THE KETOGENIC DIET

THE COMPLETE GUIDE FOR BEGINNERS

Author

Dave Robinson

Find my books on Amazon!

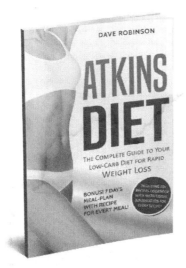

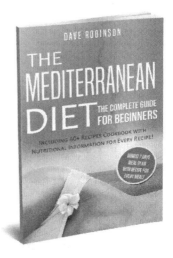

amazon.com/author/dave.robinson

Please leave feedback if you love them!

It is very important for me

TABLE OF CONTENTS

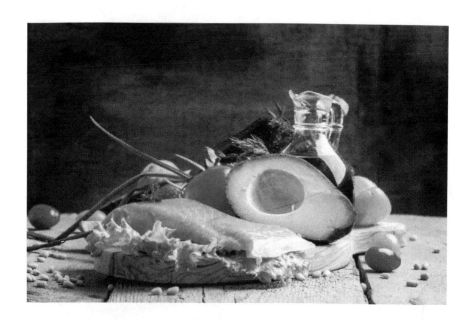

INTRODUCTION

The ketogenic diet is a special kind of diet prescribed mostly for people with epilepsy, diabetes, cancer, etc. On this diet plan, a vast change is produced in the metabolic system for the wellbeing of the patient or the client. The diet was designed by Dr. Russell Wilder in 1924 and was used at the Mayo Clinic. The metabolic change is made by switching the primary cellular fuel source from carbohydrates to fat-metabolism products called ketones. The metabolic process is called ketogenesis, while the body situation is called ketosis. In ketosis, ketones are used to make energy instead of carbohydrates. In short, this is a low-carb, high-fat diet plan. It's a very effective way to lose weight and improve one's health.

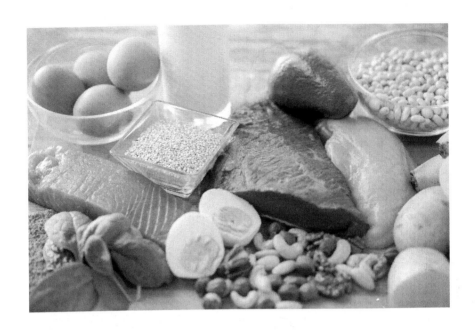

WHAT IS THE KETOGENIC DIET?

The ketogenic diet is a low-carbohydrate, high-fat, adequate-protein diet that has been implemented as a treatment for epilepsy for more than 90 years. This way of treating epilepsy was invented as an alternative to fasting, which was used for millennia to treat seizure activity. The prime feature of the ketogenic diet (aka KD) is producing ketone bodies and fatty acid oxidation in the liver, thereby reducing blood glucose levels. Ketone bodies supply a substitute which works as an alternative for energy utilization to glucose and also constitutes essential building blocks in the developing brain for the biosynthesis of lipids and cell membranes.

HISTORY OF THE KETOGENIC DIET

As a therapy for epilepsy, the ketogenic diet became popular in the 1920s and 1930s. It was introduced as an alternative to fasting, which was then mainstream. Later this therapy subsided because of the introduction of other anticonvulsant therapies. However, these medications, while effective, somehow failed to achieve significant results, controlling 20 to 30 percent of epileptics. Hence came the re-introduction of the ketogenic diet as a technique for managing the condition.

Fasting has been used in the treatment of diseases for thousands of years and was studied by Greek and Indian physicians. "On the Sacred Disease" by Hippocratic Corpus explains how altering one's diet plan plays a significant role in managing epilepsy. In his "Epidemics" collection, he also relates the story of a man who was completely cured of epilepsy by totally abstaining from food and drink.

The first modern scientific study of the ketogenic diet as a cure for epilepsy was conducted in France in 1911. Before that, potassium bromide was popular in treating epilepsy, but it slowed patients' mental capabilities. Instead, 20 patients maintained a vegetarian, low-calorie food plan that included fasting. Most patients couldn't get the diet plan but two of them showed significant improvement. As compared to taking potassium bromide, this diet plan was found to be more helpful in improving a patient's mental abilities.

In the 20th century, an American named Bernarr Macfadden made the idea of fasting popular for restoring health. His osteopath student, named Hugh Conklin, used fasting as a method to control epilepsy. He proposed that epilepsy is caused by a certain toxin secreted in the intestine and that a fast for 18 to 25 days could cause the toxin to decrease. His patients were kept on diet that resulted in the cure of 90 percent of the children and 50 percent of the adults. Thorough analysis showed that this diet made 20 percent of the patients seizure-free, while and 50 percent showed improvement. Soon, fasting became part of the treatment of epilepsy as a form of regular therapy. Dr. MacMurry told the New York Medical Journal that he had successfully treated patients of epilepsy using a diet of sugar and starch in 1912.

Rollin Woddyatt, an endocrinologist, introduced the idea that ketone bodies are made of three water-soluble compounds called acetoacetate, acetone, and b-hydroxybutyrate, which are produced by the liver if starved or following a diet rich in fat. Later, Russell Wilder from the Mayo Clinic called this diet the "ketogenic diet" and used it for epilepsy in the same year.

Additional research in the 1960s showed that more ketones are produced MCTs or medium-chain triglycerides per unit of energy and sent to the liver quickly through the hepatic portal vein opposing the lymphatic system. Peter Huttenlocher devised a ketogenic diet in 1971, showing that parents could create a more enjoyable diet for their epileptic children. This diet has been used as a regular therapy to this day.

To understand how the ketogenic diet works, we must understand how the carbohydrate diet works. Our bodies produce glucose and insulin when we eat a lot of carbs. Glucose is the easiest substance for our body to turn into energy, so it is our bodies' first choice. On the other hand, insulin is used to carry glucose around our bodies through the bloodstream. Because glucose is used as the primary energy provider, fat is stored in the body. When the intake of carbs is lowered, the body enters a situation called ketosis. It is a natural process in which our bodies start helping us thrive when food intake is low. During this process, ketones are produced from the breakdown of fats in the liver. The ketogenic diet aims to force our bodies into this situation. In this system, we are introduced to the starvation of carbohydrates, not the starvation of calories. As our bodies are very much adaptive, when we take away carbs and overload with fats, ketones are burned as the main energy resource.

Much research has been done on ketosis as it relates to various diseases. It has been proven to be not only a life-changing but also a life-saving process for people. Ketone bodies have many beneficial effects on our bodies. The ketogenic diet improves the work process of the cellular pathways as well as mitochondrial health. It is used mainly for the cure of epilepsy, as it reduces the occurrence of seizures very effectively and quickly. Children are more likely to benefit from this diet than from any anti-convulsing medicine. Again, this diet is now used to cure cancer, Alzheimer's, and autism, with the success of this cure process due mainly to the metabolic system. It is also helpful for infantile spasms, Rett syndrome, tuberous sclerosis complex, Dravet syndrome, Doose syndrome, and GLUT-1 deficiency. It is a very effective way to lose weight, too. People can use this diet blindfolded because they don't have to keep track of their calories. This diet plan is filling. One study showed that it is 2.2 time more effective than the low-fat diet. Another study showed that people on this diet lost three times more weight than those who were on Diabetes UK's recommended diet plan. Levels of triglycerides and cholesterol also improved. The ketogenic diet helps lower factors for disease. Research shows that this is, in fact, better than the low-fat diet and doctors are recommending this diet nowadays. The increased protein intake creates numerous benefits, which the increased ketones, lowered blood sugar, and insulin sensitivity play a key role in creating. It also reduces the process of lipogenesis, or the process of converting

12

sugar into fat. The best thing is that this diet gradually increases the rate of fat a person burns during work, exercise, and even rest.

The ketogenic diet is a new trend. It is a diet in which the body turns into a fat-burning machine. This diet not only helps with weight loss but is also beneficial for performance and health. However, it does have some side effects.

Generally, our diet is filled with carbs, and the main source of our energy is glucose. When we eat, our bodies turn the glucose into energy and store the fat. The ketogenic diet is focused mainly on fat. In this plan, fat is the main food intake, so the body is provided with only fat for an energy source. Thus, the body starts transforming fat into energy, cutting loose all the fats. The person starts losing weight without even trying or eating less.

Scientifically, the diet's name derives mainly from the fact that in this diet small molecules called "ketones" are produced. When blood sugar is in short supply, the body uses it as an alternative fuel. These ketones are produced when people eat very low amounts of carbs and a moderate amount of protein. Ketones are made in the liver and are used all over the body for energy. The brain is the biggest user of the energy. It can fully survive on fat or ketone. Here, the insulin level becomes very low, making it easy to access fat to burn it. However, this diet causes less hunger and a steady supply of energy.

Foods in the ketogenic diet must be eaten very cautiously. Carb-based foods like sugars, legumes, grains, rice, candy, juice, potatoes, and even fruits should be avoided.

The main food in this diet is meat (steak, sausage, chicken, red meat), eggs, fish (salmon, trout, tuna), nuts, healthy oils, low-carb veggies, avocadoes, butter, cream, unprocessed cheese (cheddar, goat, blue, cream, mozzarella), etc. Healthy herbs and spices, as well as salt and pepper, can be eaten too.

The ketogenic diet has recently gained the attention of health-conscious people. Doctors prescribe it not only for disease but for a healthy lifestyle.

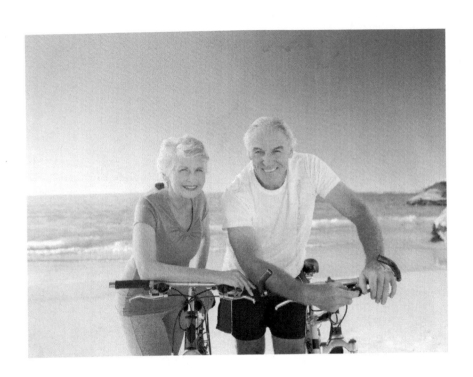

BENEFITS OF THE KETOGENIC DIET

The low-carb diet or ketosis has been a topic of controversy for a long time. People who are professionals or fat-phobic have demonized it. They have said that it will cause health issues like cholesterol or heart diseases because it is enriched with fat. However, with the advance of time, this belief has changed. Various human studies have scientifically proven that this diet is very useful for people. Not only does it promote weight loss, it also creates major improvements in cholesterol levels and other risk factors.

Here are some points that prove the benefits of the ketogenic diet:

1. Weight Loss: Today, many people successfully use the ketogenic diet for weight loss, but doctors have been prescribing

this diet for weight loss for centuries. This diet suppresses the appetite and lowers insulin levels because it lacks carbohydrates. This 1-2 combo diet is very useful in decreasing body fat levels.

2. Anti-aging: Lowered insulin levels also lower oxidative stress, which can increase one's lifespan. By lowering insulin levels, the ketogenic diet forms ketones to be used as fuel. Therefore, experts are using this diet in a quest to slow the aging process.

3. Lower Blood Sugar: The ketogenic diet allows people to utilize ketones and fat as fuel for the body. This means people with type two diabetes don't have to worry about increased blood sugar levels.

4. Cardiovascular Diseases and Metabolic Syndrome: Research has shown that, as opposed to popular belief, overweight individuals who eat a diet devoid of carbs and rich in fat may be able to reverse symptoms of cardiovascular disease.

5. Polycystic Ovary Syndrome: The ketogenic diet, because of its low carb intake and resistant insulin, can help with PCOS. This diet causes a significant change in testosterone and body weight. In a study investigating this effect, two women even became pregnant.

6. Improved Brain Function: Another thing people rave about with respect to the ketogenic diet is the improved brain function it causes. Improved learning, clarity of thought, memory recall,

etc have resulted from the ketogenic diet. Research done on rats has shown that the ketogenic diet leads to a significant improvement in performance.

7. Irritable Bowel Syndrome: Men who suffer from IBS (stomach discomfort, diarrhea, bloating, etc.) can benefit from this diet. People may be shocked by the thought of eating a low-carb, high-fat diet, and it may cause increased diarrhea in the beginning, but in the long run they will benefit.

8. Increased Mitochondrial Function: Without mitochondria, we would be dead because mitochondria are the factories that create cellular energy. Many of our bodily functions (health, energy, immune function, sports performance, etc.) depend on them. A study has shown that mitochondria work better on a ketogenic diet. They are able to increase the energy level in a steady, efficient, long-burning, and stable way. The diet also increases the energetic output of the mitochondria and lessens the creation of damaging free radicals. Mitochondria are specially designed to use fat, which decreases the toxic load and greatly increases the number of energy-producing genes.

9. Endurance: Another side effect of ketosis involves endurance, which is highly beneficial to athletes. A study has shown that those on the ketogenic diet had more mitochondria, lower oxidative stress, and a lower lactate load, which athletes on a carb diet didn't have. Also, numerous studies show that ketones in the blood lead to significant performance improvement and increased power.

10. Lowered Inflammation and Decreased Pain: The ketogenic diet helps with pain relief by reducing glucose metabolism, which can be used as a potential mechanism for action. It also has anti-inflammatory properties.

11. Stable Energy Level: Those who change from a genuine Western diet to a ketogenic diet will see their energy levels increasing and remaining stable all day long, with no cravings or mid-day slumps and without the need for instant caffeine or sugar hits. Fat is an available source of energy. When someone is fat-adapted, they can easily go hours without food and not have a problem with their energy level.

12. Less Heartburn: A study has shown that those who changed to the ketogenic diet experienced changes in less than a week. They reported that they didn't suffer from heart burn anymore. This reduction in acidity is caused by reducing carbohydrates and increasing fat content.

13. Fatty Liver Disease: As with heartburn, studies have shown that the ketogenic diet can be effective with respect to non-alcoholic fatty liver disease. Six months of the ketogenic diet has shown a significant amount of weight loss and historical improvement in fatty liver disease.

14. Migraine Treatment: Many people suffering from migraine have said that when they switched their diet from a conventional one to one that was ultra-low in carbs, they saw significant results in terms of decreasing their migraines.

15. Clean-Burning Fuel: Our bodies prefer fat as an energy source. That's why we store so many calories in the form of fat and only 200 calories in glucose form. When glucose breaks down, it creates oxygen species that are reactive as compared to fat. They are controlled by anti-oxidants. When glucose intake is lessened, carbohydrates are restricted and ketone, which is clean, is burned as a fuel instead.

16. Easier Fasting: It's easy to fast on the ketogenic diet. Those who are used to the carb diet will be shocked at the thought of not eating for 10 to 12 hours, but when you adapt to keto diet, fasting becomes very easy. You can go for a long time without food.

17. Parkinson's Disease: Ketosis has shown significant effects in improving some disease conditions, Parkinson's among them. Five individuals who went through this diet for 28 days reported that they had improved after four weeks.

18. Alzheimer's: Many studies support the idea that if the brain cannot utilize glucose, it will use ketones under the right circumstances, which will help with Alzheimer's.

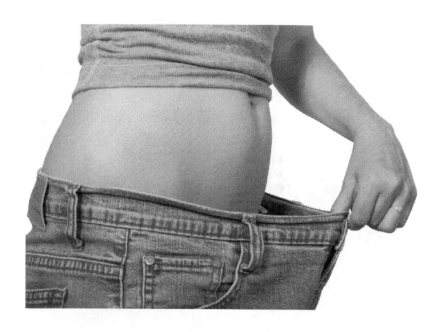

PRECAUTIONS BEFORE STARTING THE KETOGENIC DIET

In this fat-adapting diet, the body goes through a massive change. Therefore, precautions must be taken for adapting to it. Here are some tips to follow before starting the diet.

1.Drink water: This is a no-brainer and is taken for granted but trust me; it is the most difficult tip to follow. We get so caught up in our lives that we forget to stay hydrated. However, this diet system requires drinking lots and lots of water. For starters, 32 ounces of water should be consumed within the first hour of waking. Another 32 ounces of water should be consumed before noon.

2.Practice fasting: This is a great way to get into the ketogenic diet, as you are not consuming protein or carbs and reducing calories. Before starting, it's a good idea to follow a low-carb diet to avoid a hypoglycemic episode. Divide your day into two phases: the building phase and the cleansing phase. The building phase is the time between your first and last meals and the cleansing phase is the time between your last and first meals. Beginners should start with 12 to 16 hours of the cleansing phase and eight to 12 hours of the building phase. During the fast, consume herbal teas and coffee, coconut oil, and MCT oil. Also, stay hydrated. This will help stabilize sugar and boost ketone production more than just water-based fasting. Over time, when the body adapts, you may move to a four- to five-hour building phase along with an 18- to 20-hour cleansing phase each day. Maintaining ketosis will be easy if you are able to do it successfully.

3. Take in enough salts: Generally, people believe they should avoid consuming too much salt. This is due to our normal carbohydrate diet, which is enriched with salts and results in higher insulin levels. However, in the ketogenic diet, the insulin level is low, causing the kidneys to extract more salts and potentially causing an imbalance in the sodium/potassium ratio in our bodies. Therefore, you should increase your salt intake by drinking broth throughout the day, adding an extra pinch of salt to your food, or drinking one-quarter teaspoon of pink salt for every eight to 16 ounces of water.

4. Get regular exercise: Regular exercise is a very important adaptation to start the ketogenic diet, as it helps you handle the small amount of diet in your diet, which the body wants to store in the liver and muscle tissues. Exercise helps activate the glucose transport molecule, which pulls out the sugar in the blood and stores it as muscle and liver glycogen.

5. Excess protein intake is prohibited: Some people doing ketosis take in an excess amount of protein. This is dangerous because it will transform the amino acid into glucose via a

chemical system called gluconeogenesis. See how you are responding to protein if you are coming out of ketosis. The protein level is different for each person; some people do well with high protein and some do better with low. It is a good idea to get your daily protein in two or three servings, from 15 to 50 grams per meal. The lower limit applies for lower-weight individuals and the upper limit is for training males with large and strong physiques.

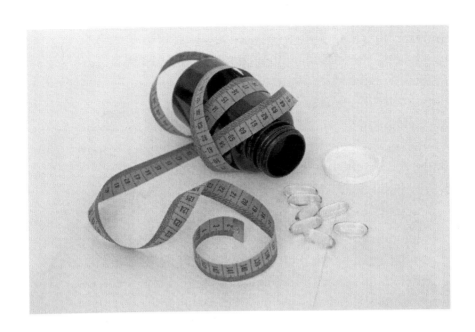

SIDE EFFECTS OF KETOSIS

Ketosis has become a new trend for quick and dramatic weight loss. However, as with any significant weight loss, as the body adapts to a new way of eating, it is normal to have some side effects. On this diet, the body switches its source of fuel from glucose to fat, which leads to side effects. Not everyone experiences these side effects, and those who do, don't experience them for long. Here are some side effects you may experience:

1.Frequent urination: At the beginning stage of ketosis, the body burns out the stored glucose in the liver and muscle. Your kidneys also begin excreting sodium in excess because of the drop in insulin level. You will have to urinate more, but once you adjust to the diet, you will be alright.

2. Dizziness and drowsiness: The body will be eliminating

minerals like magnesium, potassium, sodium, etc with the water it is getting rid of. This will make you feel lightheaded, dizzy, and fatigued. This can be avoided if you focus on eating foods rich in potassium, like broccoli, meat, poultry, dairy, fish, leafy greens, avocados, etc. Also, add salt to your food in various ways. You can have broth enriched with salts all day long; also drink water with salt dissolved in it.

3. Low blood sugar: Low blood sugar (or hypoglycemia) is another common side effect among beginners. Your body is accustomed to having a certain amount of insulin for handling the sugar in the carb diet. In the keto diet, when sugar intake is drastically lessened, hypoglycemia is possible. It can make you hungry, shaky, or tired until your body adjusts.

4. Sugar cravings: A long-term keto diet will reduce your cravings for sugar and carbs, but initially you will feel strong cravings for them. This can last from two to 21 days. Controlling it will benefit you in the long run.

5. Constipation: You may initially face some constipation as you adjust your diet. This is due to the excessive elimination of fluids from your body. To remedy this problem, drink lots of water and eat foods full of fibers and salt. Also eat non-starchy vegetables.

6. Diarrhea: Instead of constipation, some people may experience diarrhea. In response, they may make the mistake of limiting their fat intake, but don't do this. Instead, be sure your carbs are being replaced by fats instead of protein.

7. Muscle cramps: The keto diet causes muscle cramps – especially leg cramps – due to the reduced amount of salts. Like other side effects, this can be cured by drinking lots of water and eating salt, thereby reducing mineral loss and preventing cramps.

8. Keto-flu: A common side effect of the ketogenic diet among

24

beginners is a flu, called keto-flu because it shows symptoms of the "normal" flu, like headaches, lethargy, irritability, brain fog, etc. These symptoms go away completely within a few days but they can be avoided through significant water and salt intake.

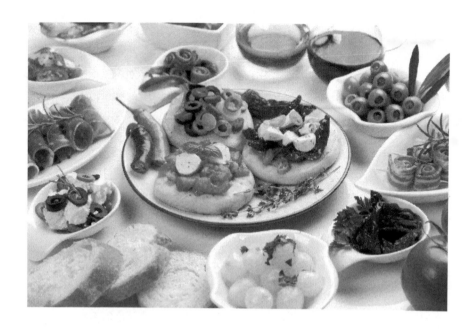

FOODS TO AVOID

Knowing what not to eat is more important in the ketogenic diet than in other diets. This is because carb- or protein-centric food may bring you out of ketosis and slow your fat-burning capabilities.

Let's take a look at the foods that should be avoided:

all white foods # CARBS:

1.Grains:All kind of grains, like wheat, oats, barley, rice, corn, rye, quinoa, sorghum, millet, bulgur, amaranth ,buckwheat, sprouted grains, etc. should be avoided because they contain a lot of carbs, which will meddle with the keto process by slowing it down.

2. Beans: Beans may be nutritious on a regular diet but they are not fit for the keto diet because they are rich in starches. Beans like black beans, chickpeas, kidney beans, lentils, lima beans, green peas, pinto beans, fava beans, etc. must be avoided.

3. Fruits: Almost all fruits and fruit-based foods like juice and smoothies are non-compliant because they are rich in sugar and carbs. If you do take in some fruits, make sure they are low in sugar, like blueberries, blackberries, and raspberries. Other fruits like pineapples, papaya, bananas, apples, oranges, mangoes, grapes, tangerines, dried fruits like dates, dried mangoes, and fruit syrups are strictly prohibited.

4. Vegetables: It is good to avoid all that grows beneath the land and to eat more leafy greens. High-starch vegetables that are rich in carbs are impediments for the keto diet. For example, yams, sweet potatoes, potatoes, carrots, parsnips, peas, yucca, corn, artichokes, cherry tomatoes, etc. are prohibited on this diet.

5. Alcohol: Vey few people can immediately sacrifice alcohol but this is important, as beer, wine, cocktails, and flavored liquors contain carbs.

PROTEINS:

Foods like sour cream, butter, yogurt, and heavy creams that are full-fat dairy are allowed on the keto diet. However, all other dairy products, like milk, low-fat cream cheese, shredded cheese, evaporated skim milk, and low-fat whipped topping must be avoided.

FAT:

All vegetable oils like soybean oil, corn oil, grapeseed oil, peanut oil, sesame oil, canola oil, and sunflower oil are very harmful to this diet.

OTHER:

Some other foods are unhealthy and harmful for this diet, like fast food, candies, margarine, sodas and soft drinks, wheat gluten, ice cream, etc because they contain extra sugar, preservatives, trans fats, etc.

SUGAR:

We often forget about the natural sugar apart from the packaged product containing added sugar. Foods like honey, maple syrup, agave nectar, raw sugar, turbinado sugar, cane sugar, and high-fructose corn syrup are threats to the keto diet.

FACTORY-FARMED PRODUCTS:

Always eat organic and grass-fed animals. Avoid grain-fed meat, factory-farmed fish, processed meat, and sausages.

ARTIFICIAL SWEETENERS:

Artificial sweeteners may seem harmless because they are not really sugar. However, they can affect the blood sugar level and cause cravings. People may react to them differently and they are known to be disruptive to ketosis. Avoid Splenda, acesulfame, Equal, aspartame, sucralose, saccharine, etc.

Condiments:

While doing keto, homemade condiments and toppings are best. If it's not possible for you to eat homemade condiments and toppings, use pure spices and herbs. If you can't do even that, avoid condiments that contain added sugar, that are made with unhealthy oils, or that are labeled "low fat."

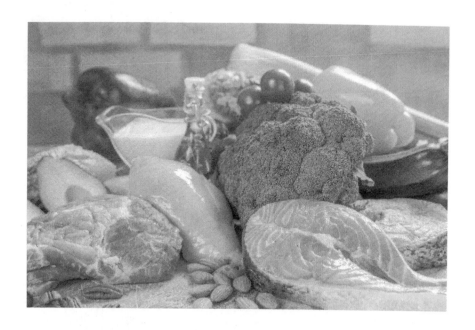

FOODS YOU CAN EAT ON THE DIET

Food intake is the most important thing on the ketogenic diet. Every food should be cautiously examined and measured. Here is a list of what you can eat on this diet:

1. Seafood: Seafood like salmon, clams, mussels, octopus, oysters, and squid is keto-friendly food because it is rich in B vitamins, potassium, and selenium and is carb-free.

2. Low-carb Veg: High in nutrients like Vitamin C and minerals and low in carbs. Non-starchy vegetables are ideal for the keto diet.

3. Cheese: There are hundreds of nutritious and delicious types of cheese that are high in fat and low in carbs – a perfect fit for the keto diet.

4. Avocados: Avocadoes are high in vitamins and minerals and very low in carbs, which is ideal for keto.

5. Poultry and Meat: If rice is a staple food of the carb diet, meat and poultry are staples of the keto diet. They are rich in high-quality protein and contain vitamins and minerals as well.

6. Eggs: Eggs are a versatile food containing less than one gram of carbs. They are high in several kinds of nutrients, which is helpful for the eyes and the heart.

DRINKS ALLOWED ON THE KETO DIET

People sometimes overlook drinks in their diet. It is very important of be cautious of drinks because many carbs come from milk, soft drinks, etc. Staying hydrated is essential on every diet. Water is the primary drink in this diet. However, drinking only water can be troublesome to some people. Here is a list of beverages to drink on this diet:

1.Sugar-free carbonated drinks: Sugar-free beverages are okay on this diet. Go for Coke Zero, Sprite Zero, Diet Coke, etc.

2. Flavored water: Not the sugar-laden varieties you'll find in shops; opt for your own flavored water. Find a suitable container and fill it with water, four or five slices of lemon, a couple slices of cucumber, a sprinkle of sweetener, a generous half-teaspoon of turmeric, ice cubes, and sprig of mint. There you go, your own flavored water.

3. Hot drinks: Trying keto-friendly hot drinks like a guilt-free hot cocoa mix with double cream and sweetener is allowed on this diet. You can also try bulletproof coffee.

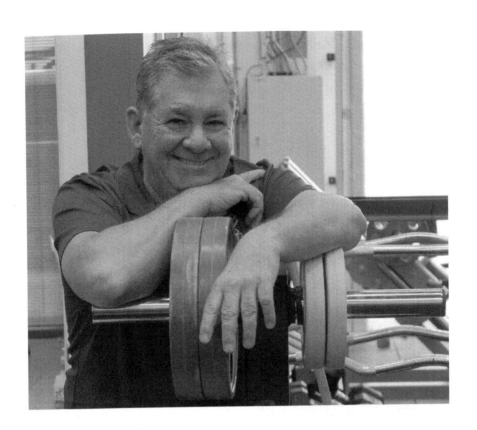

THE KETOGENIC DIET FOR MEN WHO PLAY SPORTS

It is hard to absorb this fact, but the ketogenic diet is not for everyone. However, it is quite beneficial for athletes. If they can follow the regimen carefully, they can achieve their desired result.

There are some common mistakes that high-performance people make while maintaining this diet. Let's take a look at those:

1. Afraid of fat: The ketogenic diet is very different from other general diets. Its main purpose is to activate fatty acids to work

as fuel for body strength. If he is a keto diet follower, an athlete will eat about 2900 calories a day, of which 2300 come from fat. Depending on his training, he may consume 256 grams of fat everyday because fat has nine calories per gram. For example, if one tablespoon of olive oil contains 14 grams, the athlete must consume 18 tablespoons a day.

2. Eating too much protein: Another common mistake of the beginner is that they replace carbs with protein instead of fat. This is harmful and can lead to gluconeogenesis, which is the conversion of amino acids to glucose. The glucose level must be kept low to produce ketone bodies from fatty acids.

3. Carbs coming back: This doesn't seem like a problem but it is because carbs can quickly add up, especially when you are determined to have your veggies, spices, and herbs. There are also some surprising products that contain carbs, like any processed foods, milk substitutes, salad dressings, etc.

4. Giving up too early: The ketogenic diet is a hard diet to follow. Every single cell goes through a change by switching from glucose to fat metabolism. Therefore, various side effects result, like the keto-flu, headaches, nausea, foggy brain, etc. The best thing you can do is to take things slowly and not give up in the initial stage when you are feeling off.

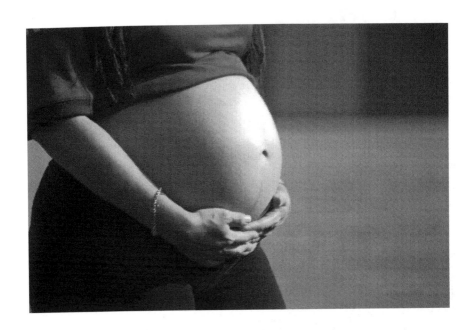

THE KETOGENIC DIET FOR WOMEN WHO ARE PREGNANT AND BREASTFEEDING

This question of whether it is safe to go keto while pregnant or breastfeeding is being asked more frequently these days. While this seems like a simple question, we must dig deeper because this simple question can have big implications!

Getting pregnant and PCOS:

One of the uses of the ketogenic diet is to cure polycystic ovary syndrome, which the diet has done with great success. From weight loss to improved hormone regulation, it's a great way to manage symptoms.

Ketosis and pregnancy:

There has been news of women getting sick from this diet while breastfeeding, but those are rare cases. Of course, it is best to always be watchful while on the keto diet. Many women and mothers have followed the keto diet without any issues and have achieved great success. However, this diet is a great demand in lactation. During lactation, the body produces carbs for breast milk. When the body doesn't get carbs through diet, it must produce them. This can put extreme pressure on the body.

The best option is to always be watchful and follow a slightly liberal low-carb program.

HOW SOON DO PEOPLE GET RESULTS ON THE KETOGENIC DIET?

When losing weight, everyone wants quick results. On the keto diet, the body is forced to use fat as fuel. The rate of weight loss varies from person to person and also varies according to the diet process. Some people may lose more than 12 pounds in a month.

When people follow the correct advice, they lose weight and lose it quickly. According to a study published in the American Journal of Clinical Nutrition in 2008, men who maintained the diet for a month lost 12 pounds on average. However, note that this was a short-term study and that results may vary.

When you lose weight too fast, you lose muscle and water

instead of fat. Health care professionals prefer a slow rate of weight loss, like one or two pounds per week. Losing weight too fast may decrease your energy levels and motivation. There is also the possibility of regaining weight. While the keto diet helps you drop weight, it's not very effective for the long term.

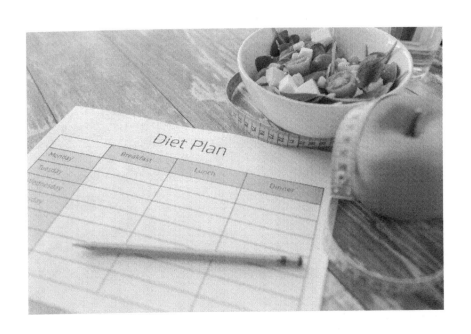

MEAL PLAN FOR 7 DAYS

	Day 1	Day 2	Day 3	Day 4	Day 5	Day 6	Day 7
Breakfast	Cream Crepes	Yogurt Waffles	Cream Cheese Pancakes	Scallion Muffins	Chives Scramble	Watercress Omelette	Spinach Quiche
Mid-morning	Turkey & Veggie Wraps	Shrimp salad	Spinach Pie	Cheese Biscuits	Devilled Eggs	Celery Crackers	Zucchini Sticks
Lunch	Avocado Salad	Beef Burger	Jalapeño Soup	Arugula salad	Cheesy Tilapia II	Broccoli Soup	Cheesy Tilapia
Mid-afternoon	Zucchini Sticks	Healthy Turkey Patties	Celery Crackers	Shrimp salad	Avocado salad	Chicken with Spinach	Cheese Biscuits
Dinner	Turkey Casserole	Beef Casserole	Chicken with Cranberries	Beef Chili	Mushroom Burger	Seafood Stew	Stuffed Leg of Lamb
Dessert	Zucchini Brownies	Cinnamon Cookies	Frozen Yoghurt	Lemon Mousse	Pumpkin Custard	Blueberry Cobbler	Strawberry Frappuccino

KETOGENIC RECIPES

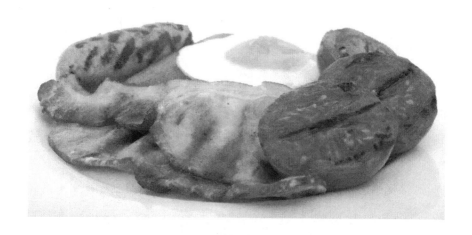

BREAKFAST RECIPES

Strawberry Smoothie

Yield: Makes 2 glasses

Ingredients

¾ cup frozen strawberries
3 tablespoons almonds, chopped
1½ cups unsweetened almond milk
2 tablespoons chia seeds
½ teaspoon ground cinnamon

Directions

1. In a high-speed blender, add all ingredients and pulse until smooth.

2. Transfer into 2 serving glasses and serve immediately.

Nutritional Information Per Serving:

Calories: 137
Fat: 9.6g
Sat. Fat: 0.8g
Sodium: 135mg
Carbohydrates: 13.4g
Fiber: 6.2g
Sugar: 3.4g
Protein: 4.2g

Cream Crepes

Yield: Makes 4 crepes (2 crepes per serving)
Cooking Time: 12 minutes

Ingredients

2 tablespoons coconut oil, melted and divided
2 organic eggs
1 teaspoon Splenda
1/8 teaspoon sea salt
2 tablespoons coconut flour
1/3 cup heavy cream

Directions

1. In a bowl, add 1 tablespoon of oil, eggs, Splenda and salt and beat until well combined. Slowly add flour, beating continuously. Add heavy cream and stir until well combined.

2. Grease a large non-stick skillet with remaining oil. Add ¼ of the mixture and tilt the pan to spread it. Cook for about 3 minutes, flipping once after 2 minutes.

3. Repeat with the remaining mixture.

Nutritional Information Per Serving:

Calories: 319
Fat: 27.4g
Sat. Fat: 19.7g
Sodium: 246mg
Carbohydrates: 10.9g
Fiber: 5.7g
Sugar: 3.4g
Protein: 8g

Cream Cheese Pancakes

Yield: Makes 4 pancakes (2 pancakes per serving)
Cooking Time: 12 minutes

Ingredients

2 organic eggs
2 ounces cream cheese, softened
½ teaspoon ground cinnamon
1 packet stevia

Directions

1. In a blender, add all the ingredients and pulse until smooth.

2. Keep aside for about 2-3 minutes.

3. Grease a large non-stick skillet with cooking spray. Add ¼ of the mixture and spread it. Cook for about 2 minutes or until golden brown. Flip and cook for about 1 minute.

4. Repeat with the remaining mixture.

Nutritional Information Per Serving:

Calories: 163
Fat: 14.3g
Sat. Fat: 7.6g
Sodium: 146mg
Carbohydrates: 2.6g
Fiber: 0.3g
Sugar: 0.4g
Protein: 7.7g

Yogurt Waffles

Yield: Makes 10 waffles (1 waffle per serving)
Cooking Time: 50 minutes

Ingredients

1 1/3 cups almond flour
2 tablespoons vanilla whey protein powder
2 tablespoons Erythritol
½ teaspoon baking soda
1 teaspoon baking powder
½ teaspoon xanthan gum
Salt, to taste
2 large organic eggs (whites and yolks separated)
2 whole organic eggs
¼ cup unsweetened almond milk
3 tablespoons butter
6 ounces Greek yogurt

Directions

1. Preheat the waffle iron and then grease it.

2. In a large bowl, add flour, protein powder, Erythritol, baking soda, baking powder, xanthan gum and salt and mix well.

3. In another small bowl, add egg whites and beat until stiff peaks form.

4. In a third medium bowl, add 2 egg yolks, whole eggs, almond milk, butter and yogurt and beat until well combined. Add egg mixture to flour mixture and mix until well combined. Gently fold in beaten egg whites.

5. Place ¼ cup of the mixture into a preheated waffle iron and cook for about 4-5 minutes or until golden brown.

6. Repeat with the remaining mixture.

Nutritional Information Per Serving:

Calories: 102
Fat: 8.5g
Sat. Fat: 36g
Sodium: 161mg
Carbohydrates: 5.4g
Fiber: 0.5g
Sugar: 4.4g
Protein: 4.9g

Scallion Muffins

Yield: Makes 12 muffins (2 muffins per serving)
Cooking Time: 30 minutes

Ingredients

½ cup almond meal
½ cup raw hemp seeds
¼ cup flaxseed meal
½ teaspoon baking powder
¼ cup nutritional yeast flakes
Salt to taste
½ cup Parmesan cheese, grated finely
½ cup low-fat cottage cheese
6 organic eggs, beaten
1/3 cup scallions, sliced thinly

Directions

1. Preheat the oven to 375 degrees F. Grease 12 cups of a small muffin tin.

2. In a large bowl, add almond meal, hemp seeds, flaxseed meal, baking powder and salt and mix well. In another bowl, add cottage cheese and eggs and mix well.

3. Add egg mixture to almond meal mixture and mix until well combined. Gently fold in scallions.

4. Transfer the mixture evenly into prepared muffin cups. Bake for about 25-30 minutes or until top becomes golden brown.

Nutritional Information Per Serving:

Calories: 306
Fat: 19.7g

Sat. Fat: 4.7g
Sodium: 398mg
Carbohydrates: 10.7g
Fiber: 4.2g
Sugar: 1.3g
Protein: 23.5g

Microwave Bread

Yield: Makes 1 Single-Serving Bread
Cooking Time: 1¼ minutes

Ingredients

1 teaspoon butter, melted
1 large organic egg
1 package Splenda
2 tablespoons flaxseed meal
½ teaspoon baking powder
¼ cup cheddar cheese, shredded

Directions

1. Coat a microwave-safe mug with 1 teaspoon melted butter.

2. In a bowl, add remaining ingredients and mix well.

3. Transfer the mixture evenly into the prepared mug.
   Microwave on high for about 1 minute. Flip the bread and
   microwave for about 10-15 seconds more.

Nutritional Information Per Serving:

Calories: 291
Fat: 23.2g
Sat. Fat: 9.9g
Sodium: 280mg
Carbohydrates: 7.7g
Fiber: 4.1g
Sugar: 0.5g
Protein: 16.4g

Zucchini Bread

Yield: Makes 1 loaf (1 slice per serving)
Cooking Time: 1 hour

Ingredients

¾ cup coconut flour
1 teaspoon baking powder
1½ teaspoons ground cinnamon
½ teaspoon salt
4 organic eggs (whites and yolks separated)
2 organic whole eggs
½ cup coconut oil, melted
½ cup unsweetened coconut milk
½ cup swerve (sugar substitute)
1 teaspoon organic vanilla extract
¾ cup zucchini, shredded

Directions

1. Preheat the oven to 350 degrees F. Grease a 9x5x3-inch bread loaf pan.

2. In a large bowl, add flour, baking powder, cinnamon and salt and mix well. In a second small bowl, add 4 egg whites and beat until fluffy.

3. In a third large bowl, add remaining ingredients except zucchini and beat until well combined.

4. Add egg mixture to the bowl with the flour mixture and mix until well combined. Fold in zucchini.

5. Gently fold in beaten egg whites.

6. Transfer the mixture evenly into the prepared loaf pan. Bake for about 1 hour or until a toothpick inserted in the

center comes out clean.

7. Remove the loaf pan from the oven and place on a wire rack to cool for at least 10-15 minutes.

8. Carefully invert the bread onto the rack to cool completely.

9. With a sharp knife, cut the loaf into slices of the desired size.

Nutritional Information Per Serving:

Calories: 74
Fat: 5.7g
Sat. Fat: 3.5g
Sodium: 159mg
Carbohydrates: 14.4g
Fiber: 0.9g
Sugar: 12.9g
Protein: 3.9g

Watercress Omelette

Yield: Makes 2 portions
Cooking Time: 5 minutes

Ingredients

2 teaspoons extra-virgin olive oil
1 cup watercress, chopped
Salt and freshly ground black pepper, to taste
4 large organic eggs, beaten
1 cup cheddar cheese, shredded

Directions

1. In a non-stick skillet, heat oil on medium-high heat. Stir in watercress and sauté for about 1 minute.

2. Stir in salt and black pepper and transfer the watercress to a bowl.

3. In the same skillet, add eggs on medium heat and cook for about 2 minutes.

4. Carefully change the side and cook for about 1 minute.

5. Place watercress over a half portion of the omelette. Sprinkle with cheese.

6. Cover the watercress and cheese with the remaining half. Cook for about 1 minute more.

7. Cut into 2 wedges and serve immediately.

Nutritional Information Per Serving:

Calories: 414
Fat: 33.4g
Sat. Fat: 15.7g

Sodium: 579mg
Carbohydrates: 1.6g
Fiber: 1.9g
Sugar: 1.1g
Protein: 27.2g

Chives Scramble

Yield: Makes 6 portions
Cooking Time: 10 minutes

Ingredients

2 tablespoons unsalted butter
1 jalapeño pepper, chopped
1 small red onion, chopped
12 large organic eggs, beaten lightly
Salt and freshly ground black pepper, to taste
2 tablespoons chives, chopped finely
4 ounces goat cheese, crumbled

Directions

1. In a large skillet, melt butter on medium heat. Add jalapeño pepper and onion and sauté for about 4-5 minutes.

2. Add eggs, salt and black pepper and cook for about 3 minutes, stirring continuously.

3. Remove from heat and immediately stir in chives and cheese.

4. Serve immediately.

Nutritional Information Per Serving:

Calories: 268
Fat: 20.5g
Sat. Fat: 10.2g
Sodium: 260mg
Carbohydrates: 2.5g
Fiber: 0.4g
Sugar: 1.8g
Protein: 18.6g

Spinach Quiche

Yield: Makes 6 portions
Cooking Time: 38 minutes

Ingredients

1 tablespoon olive oil
1 onion, chopped
1 (10-ounce) package frozen spinach, thawed
3 cups Muenster cheese, shredded
5 organic eggs, beaten
Salt and freshly ground black pepper, to taste

Directions

1. Preheat the oven to 350 degrees F. Lightly grease a 9-inch pie dish.

2. In a large skillet, heat oil on medium heat. Add onion and sauté for about 4-5 minutes. Increase the heat to medium high.

3. Add spinach and cook for about 2-3 minutes or until all the liquid is absorbed. Remove from the heat and set aside to cool slightly.

4. In a large bowl, mix the remaining ingredients. Add the spinach mixture and stir to combine.

5. Transfer the mixture into the prepared pie dish. Bake for about 30 minutes.

6. Remove from the oven and set aside to cool for about 10 minutes before serving.

7. Cut into 6 equal-sized wedges and serve.

Nutritional Information Per Serving:

Calories: 299
Fat: 23.1g
Sat. Fat: 12.3g
Sodium: 471mg
Carbohydrates: 4.4g
Fiber: 1.4g
Sugar: 1.9g
Protein: 19.4g

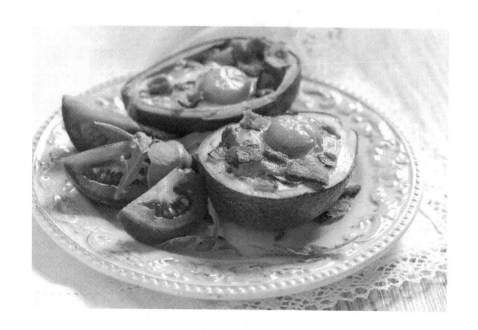

LUNCH RECIPES

Arugula Salad

Yield: Makes 2 plates

Ingredients

¼ cup fresh basil, chopped
1 garlic clove, minced
2 tablespoons extra-virgin olive oil
1 tablespoon balsamic vinegar
Salt and freshly ground black pepper, to taste
2 medium ripe tomatoes, cut into slices
3 ounces Mozzarella cheese, cubed
3 cups arugula

Directions

1. In a small blender, add basil, garlic, olive oil, vinegar, a pinch of salt and fresh cracked pepper and pulse until smooth.

2. In a large serving bowl, mix remaining ingredients. Pour dressing and toss to coat well.

3. Serve immediately.

Nutritional Information Per Serving:

Calories: 274
Fat: 22g
Sat. Fat: 6.6g
Sodium: 347mg
Carbohydrates: 8.1g
Fiber: 2.1g
Sugar: 3.9g
Protein: 14.1g

Avocado Salad

Yield: Makes 4 plates

Ingredients

For Salad:

2 medium avocados, peeled, pitted and sliced
6 cups fresh spinach leaves, torn
1 cup blue cheese, crumbled
¼ cup almonds, toasted and chopped

For Dressing:

1½ tablespoons balsamic vinegar
3 tablespoons extra-virgin olive oil
1 teaspoon unsweetened applesauce
Salt and freshly ground black pepper, to taste

Directions

1. In a large serving bowl, add all salad ingredients except almonds and mix.

2. In another bowl, add all dressing ingredients and beat until well combined. Pour dressing over salad and gently toss to coat well.

3. Serve immediately, topping with almonds.

Nutritional Information Per Serving:

Calories: 314
Fat: 28.6g
Sat. Fat: 8.8g
Sodium: 548mg
Carbohydrates: 6.9g

Fiber: 4.2g
Sugar: 1g
Protein: 10.5g

Broccoli Soup

Yield: Makes 4 bowls
Cooking Time: 15 minutes

Ingredients

4 cups low-sodium chicken broth
20 ounces small broccoli florets
12 ounces cheddar cheese, cubed
Freshly ground black pepper, to taste
1 cup heavy cream

Directions

1. In a large soup pan, add broth and broccoli and bring to a boil on medium-high heat.

2. Reduce the heat to low and simmer, covered, for about 5-7 minutes.

3. Stir in cheese and simmer for about 2-3 minutes, stirring until cheese is melted completely.

4. Stir in black pepper and cream and simmer for about 2 minutes. Serve hot.

Nutritional Information Per Serving:

Calories: 340
Fat: 26.5g
Sat. Fat: 16.6g
Sodium: 438mg
Carbohydrates: 8.2g
Fiber: 2.5g
Sugar: 1.9g
Protein: 18.5g

Jalapeño Soup

Yield: Makes 5 bowls
Cooking Time: 35 minutes

Ingredients

8 bacon slices, chopped
4 medium jalapeño peppers, seeded and chopped
¼ cup unsalted butter
1 teaspoon dried thyme, crushed
½ teaspoon ground cumin
3 cups low-sodium chicken broth
8 ounces cheddar cheese, shredded
¾ cup heavy cream
Freshly ground black pepper, to taste

Directions

1. Heat a non-stick skillet on medium heat. Add bacon and cook for about 8-10 minutes or until crisp. Transfer the bacon onto a paper-towel-lined plate, reserving the grease in the skillet.

2. In the same skillet, add jalapeño peppers and sauté for about 1-2 minutes. Transfer the jalapeño peppers onto the plate with the bacon.

3. Transfer the remaining bacon grease into a large soup pan. Add butter and heat on medium. Add spices and sauté for about 1 minute.

4. Add broth and bring to a boil. Reduce the heat to low and simmer for about 15 minutes. Remove from heat and with an immersion blender, blend until well combined.

5. Return the pan to medium-low heat. Stir in half of the cooked bacon, cooked jalapeño, cheese, cream and black

pepper and simmer for about 5 minutes.

6. Serve hot with the topping of remaining bacon.

Nutritional Information Per Serving:

Calories: 592
Fat: 50.5g
Sat. Fat: 26g
Sodium: 1762mg
Carbohydrates: 3.4g
Fiber: 0.6g
Sugar: 0.7g
Protein: 30.4g

Cheesy Spinach

Yield: Makes 4 portions
Cooking Time: 15 minutes

Ingredients

2 tablespoons unsalted butter
1 medium onion, chopped
1 cup cream cheese, softened
2 (10-ounce) packages frozen spinach, thawed and squeezed dry
2-3 tablespoons water
Pinch of salt
Freshly ground black pepper, to taste
2 teaspoons fresh lemon juice

Directions

1. In a skillet, melt butter on medium heat. Add onion and sauté for about 6-8 minutes.

2. Add the cream cheese and cook for about 2 minutes until melted completely. Stir in spinach and water and cook for about 4-5 minutes.

3. Stir in salt, black pepper and lemon juice and remove from heat.

4. Serve immediately.

Nutritional Information Per Serving:

Calories: 298
Fat: 26.6g
Sat. Fat: 16.5g
Sodium: 365mg
Carbohydrates: 9.3g
Fiber: 3.7g
Sugar: 1.9g
Protein: 8.8g

Cheesy Cauliflower

Yield: Makes 5 portions
Cooking Time: 30 minutes

Ingredients

1 head cauliflower
1 tablespoon prepared mustard
1 teaspoon mayonnaise
¼ cup butter, cut into small pieces
½ cup Parmesan cheese, grated

Directions

1. Preheat the oven to 375 degrees F.

2. In a bowl, mix mustard and mayonnaise. Coat the cauliflower head with the mustard mixture.

3. Arrange the cauliflower head in a baking dish. Top the cauliflower with the butter in the shape of dots.

4. Sprinkle evenly with cheese. Bake for about 30 minutes.

5. Serve hot.

Nutritional Information Per Serving:

Calories: 167
Fat: 14.1g
Sat. Fat: 8.7g
Sodium: 395mg
Carbohydrates: 3.8g
Fiber: 1.4g
Sugar: 1.4g
Protein: 7.4g

Creamy Brussels Sprout

Yield: Makes 5 portions
Cooking Time: 20 minutes

Ingredients

1½ pounds fresh Brussels sprouts, trimmed and halved
3 garlic cloves, minced
2 tablespoons butter, melted
2 tablespoons Dijon mustard
½ cup heavy whipping cream
Salt and freshly ground white pepper, to taste

Directions

1. Preheat the oven to 450 degrees F.

2. In a large roasting pan, add Brussels sprouts, garlic and butter and toss to coat well. Roast for about 10-15 minutes, tossing occasionally.

3. In a small pan, add remaining ingredients on medium-low heat and bring to a gentle boil. Cook for about 1-2 minutes, stirring continuously.

4. Serve Brussels sprouts with the topping of creamy sauce.

Nutritional Information Per Serving:

Calories: 148
Fat: 9.8g
Sat. Fat: 5.9g
Sodium: 174mg
Carbohydrates: 13.6g
Fiber: 5.4g
Sugar: 3g
Protein: 5.3g

Green Beans with Tomatoes

Yield: Makes 8 portions
Cooking Time: 40 minutes

Ingredients

¼ teaspoon fresh lemon peel, grated finely
2 teaspoons butter, melted
Salt and freshly ground white pepper, to taste
4 cups grape tomatoes
1½ pounds fresh green beans, trimmed
½ cup Parmesan cheese, grated

Directions

1. Preheat the oven to 350 degrees F.

2. In a large bowl, mix lemon peel, butter, salt and white pepper.

3. Add cherry tomatoes and toss to coat well. Transfer the tomato mixture into a roasting pan.

4. Roast for about 35-40 minutes, stirring once halfway through.

5. Ina pan of boiling water, arrange a steamer basket. Place green beans in the basket.

6. Cover and steam for about 7-8 minutes. Drain well.

7. Divide the green beans and tomatoes on serving plates. Sprinkle with cheese and serve.

Nutritional Information Per Serving:

Calories: 110
Fat: 5.9g

Sat. Fat: 3.6g
Sodium: 219mg
Carbohydrates: 9.9g
Fiber: 4g
Sugar: 3.6g
Protein: 6.2g

Green Beans with Mushrooms

Yield: Makes 4 portions
Cooking Time: 25 minutes

Ingredients

2 tablespoons butter
2 tablespoons onion, minced
½ teaspoon garlic, minced
1 (8-ounce) package white mushrooms, sliced
2 cooked bacon slices, crumbled
Pinch of salt
1 cup frozen green beans

Directions

1. In a large skillet, melt butter on medium heat. Add onion and garlic and sauté for about 1 minute.

2. Add mushrooms and cook for about 5 minutes.

3. Stir in bacon and salt and cook for about 5-10 minutes. Stir in green beans and cook for about 5-10 minutes more.

4. Serve hot.

Nutritional Information Per Serving:

Calories: 153
Fat: 12g
Sat. Fat: 5.7g
Sodium: 429mg
Carbohydrates: 4.6g
Fiber: 1.6g
Sugar: 1.6g
Protein: 7.8g

Veggie Combo

Yield: Makes 6 portions
Cooking Time: 25 minutes

Ingredients

4 bacon slices
1 pound frozen okra, thawed, trimmed and sliced
½ green bell pepper, seeded and chopped
2 celery stalks, chopped
1 small onion, chopped
2 cups tomatoes, chopped finely
Salt and freshly ground black pepper, to taste

Directions

1. Heat a large non-stick skillet on medium-high heat.

2. Add bacon and cook for about 8-10 minutes or until crisp.

3. Transfer the bacon into a bowl, reserving fats in the skillet. Crumble the bacon and set aside.

4. In the same skillet, add okra, celery and onion and sauté for about 5-6 minutes

5. . Stir in tomatoes, salt and black pepper and cook for about 3-4 minutes.

6. Serve hot with the topping of bacon.

Nutritional Information Per Serving:

Calories: 154
Fat: 8.4g
Sat. Fat: 2.7g
Sodium: 487mg

Carbohydrates: 10.3g
Fiber: 3.6g
Sugar: 3.8g
Protein: 9.4g

Turkey & Veggie Wraps

Yield: Makes 10 wraps (1 wrap per serving)
Cooking Time: 15 minutes

Ingredients

2 tablespoons unsalted butter
1 pound lean ground turkey
1 onion, chopped
2 garlic cloves, minced
1 green bell pepper, seeded and chopped
1 cup carrots, peeled and chopped
½ cup summer squash, chopped
½ cup zucchini, chopped
2 tablespoons low-sodium soy sauce
½ teaspoon curry powder
Freshly ground black pepper, to taste
10 large lettuce leaves
1½ cups Parmesan cheese, shredded

Directions

1. In a large skillet, melt butter on medium heat.

2. Add turkey and cook for about 4-5 minutes, breaking the lumps.

3. Add vegetables and cook for about 4-5 minutes. Add soy sauce, curry powder and black pepper and cook for about 4-5 minutes.

4. Arrange lettuce leaves onto serving plates.

5. Divide the turkey mixture evenly over the leaves.

6. Sprinkle with cheese and serve.

Nutritional Information Per Serving:

Calories: 136
Fat: 7.8g
Sat. Fat: 2.6g
Sodium: 372mg
Carbohydrates: 4.3g
Fiber: 0.9g
Sugar: 2.2g
Protein: 12.7g

Mushroom Burgers

Yield: Makes 4 burgers (1 burger per serving)
Cooking Time: 16 minutes

Ingredients

¼ cup balsamic vinegar
2 tablespoons olive oil
½ teaspoon dried oregano, crushed
½ teaspoon dried basil, crushed
Salt and freshly ground black pepper, to taste
4 Portobello mushroom caps, stems removed
4 (1-ounce) provolone cheese slices
4 tomato slices
2 tablespoons fresh basil leaves

Directions

1. Preheat the grill to medium-high heat. Grease the grill grate.

2. In a small bowl, mix the vinegar, oil, herbs, salt and pepper. In a shallow dish, arrange the mushroom caps, smooth side up.

3. Place the oil mixture over the mushroom caps and set aside for about 15 minutes.

4. Remove the mushroom caps from the bowl, reserving the marinade.

5. Grill the mushroom caps for about 5-8 minutes per side, occasionally basting with the reserved marinade.

6. In the last 2 minutes of cooking, arrange 1 cheese slice over each mushroom cap.

7. Top each burger with 1 tomato slice and basil and serve.

Nutritional Information Per Serving:

Calories: 190
Fat: 15.3g
Sat. Fat: 6.1g
Sodium: 162mg
Carbohydrates: 6.2g
Fiber: 1.6g
Sugar: 2g
Protein: 9.4g

Tuna Burgers

Yield: Makes 2 burgers (1 burger per serving)
Cooking Time: 6 minutes

Ingredients

1 (15-ounce) can water-packed tuna, drained
½ celery stalk, chopped
2 tablespoons fresh parsley, copped
1 teaspoon fresh dill, chopped
2 tablespoons walnuts, chopped
2 tablespoons mayonnaise
1 organic egg, beaten
1 tablespoon butter
¼ cup cheddar cheese, shredded

Directions

1. In a bowl, add all ingredients except butter and cheese and mix until well combined.

2. Make 2 equal-sized patties from the mixture.

3. In a frying pan, melt butter on medium heat. Add patties and cook for about 2-3 minutes.

4. Carefully flip, then top each patty evenly with cheese. Cook for about 2-3 minutes.

5. Serve hot.

Nutritional Information Per Serving:

Calories: 644
Fat: 39.4g
Sat. Fat: 11.8g
Sodium: 377mg

Carbohydrates: 5.3g
Fiber: 0.8g
Sugar: 1.4g
Protein: 65g

Beef Burgers

Yield: Makes 2 burgers (1 burger per serving)
Cooking Time: 5 minutes

Ingredients

8 ounces lean ground beef
Salt and freshly ground black pepper, to taste
1 ounce Mozzarella cheese, cubed
1 tablespoon butter
2 ounces cheddar cheese, sliced
2 cooked bacon slices, chopped

Directions

1. In a bowl, add all ingredients except butter and cheese and mix until well combined.

2. Make 2 equal-sized patties from the mixture. Place mozzarella cubes inside each patty and cover with the beef.

3. In a frying pan, melt butter on medium heat. Add patties and cook for about 2-3 minutes. Carefully flip, then top each patty evenly with cheese. Cook for about 1-2 minutes.

4. Serve hot with the topping of bacon.

Nutritional Information Per Serving:

Calories: 573
Fat: 36.9g
Sat. Fat: 17.8g
Sodium: 1047mg
Carbohydrates: 1.3g
Fiber: 0g
Sugar: 0.2g
Protein: 56.3g

Buttered Scallops

Yield: Makes 2 portions
Cooking Time: 5 minutes

Ingredients

¼ cup butter
2 tablespoons fresh rosemary, chopped
2 garlic cloves, minced
1 pound sea scallops

Directions

1. In a medium skillet, melt butter on medium-high heat. Add rosemary and garlic and sauté for about 1 minute.

2. Add scallops and cook for about 2 minutes each side or until desired doneness.

3. Serve hot.

Nutritional Information Per Serving:

Calories: 272
Fat: 16.8g
Sat. Fat: 10g
Sodium: 354mg
Carbohydrates: 5.7g
Fiber: 1g
Sugar: 0g
Protein: 25.8g

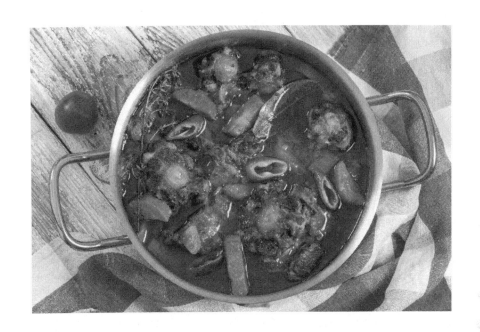

DINNER RECIPES

Steak & Plum Salad

Yield: Makes 4 plates
Cooking Time: 10 minutes

Ingredients

4 teaspoons fresh lemon juice, divided
1½ tablespoons olive oil
Salt and freshly ground black pepper, to taste
1 pound grass-fed flank steak, trimmed
1 teaspoon honey
8 cups baby arugula
3 plums, pitted and sliced thinly
¼ cup blue cheese, crumbled

Directions:

1. In a large bowl, mix 1 teaspoon of lemon juice, 1½ teaspoons of olive oil, salt and black pepper. Add steak and coat generously with mixture.

2. Heat a greased non-stick skillet on medium-high heat. Add beef steak and cook for about 5 minutes per side.

3. Transfer the steak onto a cutting board. Keep aside for about 10 minutes before slicing.

4. With a sharp knife, cut the beef steak diagonally across the grain in the desired-sized slices.

5. In a large bowl, add the remaining lemon juice, oil, honey, salt and black pepper and beat well.

6. Add arugula and toss well.

7. Divide arugula in 4 serving plates.

8. Top evenly with beef slices, plum slices and cheese and serve.

Nutritional Information Per Serving:

Calories: 329
Fat: 17.6g
Sat. Fat: 6.3g
Sodium: 232mg
Carbohydrates: 7.9g
Fiber: 1.4g
Sugar: 6.4g
Protein: 34.8g

Shrimp Salad

Yield: Makes 12 plates
Cooking Time: 5 minutes

Ingredients

4 pounds large shrimp
1 lemon, quartered
3 cups celery stalks, chopped
1 red onion, chopped
2 cups mayonnaise
2 tablespoons balsamic vinegar
1 teaspoon Dijon mustard
Salt and freshly ground black pepper, to taste

Directions:

1. In a large pan of salted boiling water, add shrimp and lemon and cook for about 3 minutes.

2. Drain well and set aside to cool. Peel and devein the shrimps.

3. In a large bowl, add cooked shrimp and all remaining ingredients. Gently stir to combine.

4. Serve immediately.

Nutritional Information Per Serving:

Calories: 342
Fat: 15.7g
Sat. Fat: 2.7g
Sodium: 673mg
Carbohydrates: 13.7g
Fiber: 0.7g
Sugar: 3.3g
Protein: 35.1g

Meatball Soup

Yield: Makes 6 bowls
Cooking Time: 5 minutes

Ingredients

For Meatballs

1 pound lean ground turkey
1 garlic clove, minced
1 organic egg, beaten
¼ cup Parmesan cheese, grated
Pinch of salt
Freshly ground black pepper, to taste

For Soup

1 tablespoon oil
1 small onion, chopped finely
1 garlic clove, minced
6 cups low-sodium chicken broth
8 cups fresh kale, trimmed and chopped
2 organic eggs, beaten lightly
¼ cup Parmesan cheese, grated
Freshly ground black pepper, to taste

Directions:

1. In a bowl, add all meatball ingredients and mix until well combined. Make equal-sized small balls from the mixture.

2. In a large soup pan, heat oil on medium heat. Add onion and sauté for about 5-6 minutes.

3. Add garlic and sauté for about 1 minute.

4. Add broth and bring to a boil. Carefully place the balls in

the pan and bring to a boil.

5. Reduce the heat to low and simmer for about 10 minutes.

6. Stir in kale and bring the soup to a gentle simmer. Simmer for about 2-3 minutes.

7. Slowly add beaten eggs, stirring continuously. Stir in cheese until melted.

8. Season with salt and black pepper and serve hot.

Nutritional Information Per Serving:

Calories: 280
Fat: 13.5g
Sat. Fat: 5g
Sodium: 424mg
Carbohydrates: 12.4g
Fiber: 1.6g
Sugar: 0.7g
Protein: 27.5g

Chicken Soup

Yield: Makes 6 bowls
Cooking Time: 35 minutes

Ingredients

2 tablespoons butter
1 medium carrot, peeled and chopped
½ cup onions, chopped
2 celery stalks, chopped
1 garlic clove, minced
2 teaspoons xanthan gum
1 teaspoon dried parsley, crushed
1 teaspoon freshly ground black pepper
4 cups low-sodium chicken broth
12 ounces cauliflower, chopped
2 cups cooked chicken, chopped
2 cups heavy cream
¼ cup fresh parsley, chopped

Directions:

1. In a large soup pan, melt butter on medium heat. Add carrot, onion and celery and sauté for about 4-5 minutes.

2. Add garlic and sauté for about 1 minute.

3. In a bowl, mix xanthan gum, parsley and black pepper. Sprinkle the soup with the parsley mixture and stir to combine.

4. Add broth and cauliflower and bring to a boil.

5. Reduce the heat to low and simmer, covered, for about 20 minutes, stirring occasionally.

6. Stir in cooked chicken, cream, parsley and salt and simmer

for about 3-4 minutes.

7. Serve hot.

Nutritional Information Per Serving:

Calories: 280
Fat: 20.2g
Sat. Fat: 12.1g
Sodium: 171mg
Carbohydrates: 8g
Fiber: 2.7g
Sugar: 2.4g
Protein: 17.2g

Seafood Stew

Yield: Makes 8 bowls
Cooking Time: 30 minutes

Ingredients

1 tablespoon olive oil
1 medium onion, chopped finely
1½ teaspoons garlic, minced and divided
¼ teaspoon red pepper flakes, crushed
1 teaspoon fresh lemon peel, grated finely
½ pound plum tomatoes, seeded and chopped finely
1 tablespoon sugar-free tomato paste
2 cups low-sodium chicken broth
1 pound red snapper fillets, cubed into 1-inch size
1 pound raw large shrimp, peeled and deveined
½ pound sea scallops
1/3 cup fresh parsley, chopped finely
½ cup mayonnaise

Directions:

1. In a large pan, heat oil on medium heat.

2. Add onion and sauté for about 4-6 minutes.

3. Add ½ teaspoon of garlic and red pepper flakes and sauté for about 1 minute.

4. Add lemon peel and tomatoes and cook, stirring for about 2-3 minutes.

5. Add tomato paste, broth and salt and bring to a boil. Reduce the heat to low and simmer, covered, for about 10 minutes.

6. Stir in seafood and parsley and simmer, covered, for about

8-10 minutes or until desired doneness.

7. Remove from heat and transfer the stew into serving bowls. In a small bowl, mix the remaining garlic and mayonnaise.

8. Top the stew evenly with garlic mayo and serve.

Nutritional Information Per Serving:

Calories: 255
Fat: 8.9g
Sat. Fat: 1.5g
Sodium: 329mg
Carbohydrates: 9g
Fiber: 0.8g
Sugar: 3g
Protein: 33.5g

Beef Chili

Yield: Makes 8 bowls
Cooking Time: 3 hours, 10 minutes

Ingredients

2 pounds grass-fed ground beef
1 onion, chopped
½ cup green bell pepper, seeded and chopped
½ cup carrot, peeled and chopped
4 ounces fresh mushrooms, sliced
2 garlic cloves, minced
1 (6-ounce) can sugar-free tomato paste
2 tablespoons red chili powder
1 tablespoon ground cumin
1 teaspoon ground cinnamon
1 teaspoon red pepper flakes, crushed
½ teaspoon ground allspice
Salt and freshly ground black pepper, to taste
4 cups water
1 cup sour cream

Directions

1. Heat a large non-stick pan on medium-high heat.

2. Add beef and cook for about 8-10 minutes.

3. Drain the excess grease from the pan. Stir in the remaining ingredients except the sour cream and bring to a boil.

4. Reduce the heat to low and simmer, covered, for about 3 hours.

5. Serve hot with the topping of sour cream.

Nutritional Information Per Serving:

Calories: 315
Fat: 13.8g
Sat. Fat: 6.5g
Sodium: 161mg
Carbohydrates: 10.3g
Fiber: 2.6g
Sugar: 4.4g
Protein: 37.4g

Chicken with Cranberries

Yield: Makes 5 portions
Cooking Time: 15 minutes

Ingredients

2 tablespoons unsalted butter, divided
1½ pound grass-fed skinless, boneless chicken thighs
Freshly ground black pepper, to taste
¼ cup onions, chopped finely
2 tablespoons fresh ginger, minced
1 cup low-sodium chicken broth
1 tablespoon fresh lemon juice
1 cup fresh cranberries
2 tablespoons unsweetened applesauce

Directions:

1. In a large skillet, melt 1 tablespoon of butter on medium heat.

2. Add the chicken and sprinkle with salt and black pepper.

3. Cook for about 5 minutes per side. Transfer the chicken into a large bowl and cover with foil to keep warm.

4. In the same skillet, add onion on medium heat and sauté for about 2-3 minutes.

5. Add chicken broth and bring to a boil, stirring occasionally to loosen the brown bits of skillet. Stir in cranberries and cook for about 5 minutes.

6. Stir in desired applesauce, salt and black pepper and cook for about 1-2 minutes.

7. Stir in remaining butter and remove from heat.

8. Pour cranberry mixture over chicken and serve.

Nutritional Information Per Serving:

Calories: 199
Fat: 8g
Sat. Fat: 4g
Sodium: 81mg
Carbohydrates: 4.2g
Fiber: 1.16g
Sugar: 1.5g
Protein: 25.9g

Chicken with Spinach

Yield: Makes 4 portions
Cooking Time: 15 minutes

Ingredients

2 tablespoons butter, divided
1 pound grass-fed chicken tenders
Salt and freshly ground black pepper, to taste
2 garlic cloves, minced
10 ounces frozen chopped spinach, thawed
¼ cup Parmesan cheese, shredded
¼ cup heavy cream

Directions:

1. In a large skillet, melt 1 tablespoon of butter on medium-high heat.

2. Add chicken and sprinkle with salt and black pepper. Cook for about 2 minutes from both sides.

3. Transfer the chicken into a bowl.

4. In the same skillet, melt the remaining butter on medium-low heat.

5. Add garlic and sauté for about 1 minute. Add spinach and cook for about 1 minute.

6. Add cheese, cream, salt and black pepper and stir to combine.

7. Spread the spinach mixture in the bottom of the skillet evenly. Place the chicken over the spinach in a single layer.

8. Immediately reduce the heat to low and simmer, covered, for about 5 minutes or until desired doneness of chicken.

9. Serve hot.

Nutritional Information Per Serving:

Calories: 394
Fat: 22.7g
Sat. Fat: 11.2g
Sodium: 575mg
Carbohydrates: 4g
Fiber: 1.6g
Sugar: 0.3g
Protein: 42.7g

Creamy Turkey Breast

Yield: Makes 14 portions
Cooking Time: 2½ hours

Ingredients

2 garlic cloves, minced
Salt and freshly ground black pepper, to taste
1 (7-pound) bone-in turkey breast
1½ cups Italian dressing

Directions:

1. Preheat the oven to 325 degrees F. Grease a 13x9-inch baking dish.

2. In a bowl, mix the seasoning. Rub the turkey breast with the seasoning mixture.

3. Arrange the turkey breast in the baking dish. Top evenly with Italian dressing.

4. Bake for about 2-2½ hours, coating occasionally with pan juices.

Nutritional Information Per Serving:

Calories: 459
Fat: 23.3g
Sat. Fat: 5.2g
Sodium: 303mg
Carbohydrates: 2.8g
Fiber: 0g
Sugar: 2.1g
Protein: 48.7g

Turkey Casserole

Yield: Makes 8 portions
Cooking Time: 1 hour

Ingredients

2 medium zucchinis, sliced
2 medium tomatoes, sliced
¾ pound ground turkey
1 large onion, chopped
2 medium garlic cloves, minced
1 cup sugar-free tomato sauce
½ cup cheddar cheese, shredded
2 cups cottage cheese, shredded
1 organic egg yolk
1 tablespoon fresh rosemary, minced
Salt and freshly ground black pepper, to taste

Directions:

1. Preheat the oven to 500 degrees F. Grease a large roasting pan

2. Arrange zucchini and tomato slices into prepared roasting pan. Spray with cooking spray.

3. Roast for about 10-12 minutes. Remove from oven.

4. Meanwhile, heat a non-stick skillet on medium-high heat. Add turkey and cook for about 4-5 minutes or until browned.

5. Add onion and garlic and cook for about 4-5 minutes.

6. Stir in tomato sauce and cook for about 2-3 minutes.

7. Reduce the temperature of the oven to 350 degrees F.

8. Transfer the turkey mixture into a 13x9-inch shallow baking dish. Place the roasted vegetables over the turkey mixture. In a bowl, mix the remaining ingredients. Spread the cheese mixture evenly over the vegetables. Bake for about 35 minutes.

9. Cut into 9 equal-sized slices and serve.

Nutritional Information Per Serving:

Calories: 209
Fat: 9g
Sat. Fat: 3.2g
Sodium: 507mg
Carbohydrates: 9g
Fiber: 2g
Sugar: 4g
Protein: 23g

Beef Casserole

Yield: Makes 8 portions
Cooking Time: 1 hour, 15 minutes

Ingredients

6 bacon slices, chopped
2 pounds ground beef
½ cup onion, chopped
Salt and freshly ground black pepper, to taste
8 ounces cheddar cheese, shredded and divided
1 organic egg, beaten
16 ounces frozen green beans
3 tablespoons butter, divided
16 ounces frozen cauliflower
¼ cup sour cream

Directions:

1. Preheat the oven to 350 degrees F. Lightly grease a baking dish.

2. Heat a large non-stick skillet on medium-high heat. Add bacon and cook for about 8-10 minutes or until crisp.

3. Drain the excess fats and transfer the bacon into a bowl.

4. In the same skillet, add beef and cook for about 4-5 minutes.

5. Add onion and cook for about 4-5 minutes. Drain the excess fats. Stir in salt and black pepper and remove from heat.

6. Stir in ½ of cheese, egg and cooked bacon and transfer into a baking dish.

7. In a pan of boiling water, add green beans and cook for

about 4-5 minutes.

8. Drain well and transfer into a bowl. Add 1 tablespoon of butter and some salt and mix.

9. In the same pan, add cauliflower and boil for about 10-12 minutes. Drain well.

10. In a food processor, add cauliflower, sour cream, the remaining butter and a pinch of salt and black pepper. Pulse until smooth.

11. Place green beans evenly over beef mixture. Top evenly with cauliflower mixture.

12. Sprinkle evenly with remaining cheese. Bake for about 35 minutes or until bubbly.

Nutritional Information Per Serving:

Calories: 500
Fat: 29.1g
Sat. Fat: 14.5g
Sodium: 668mg
Carbohydrates: 8.7g
Fiber: 3.5g
Sugar: 2.7g
Protein: 50g

Stuffed Leg of Lamb

Yield: Makes 12 portions
Cooking Time: 1 hour, 45 minutes

Ingredients

1/3 cup fresh parsley, minced finely
8 garlic cloves, minced and divided
3 tablespoons extra-virgin olive oil, divided
Salt and freshly ground black pepper, to taste
1 (4-pound) boneless leg of lamb, butterflied and trimmed
1/3 cup red onion, minced
4 cups fresh kale, trimmed and chopped
½ cup kalamata olives, pitted and chopped
½ cup feta cheese, crumbled
1 teaspoon fresh lemon zest, grated finely

Directions:

1. In a large baking dish, mix parsley, 4 garlic cloves, 2 tablespoons of oil, salt and black pepper.

2. Add leg of lamb and coat generously with parsley mixture. Set aside at room temperature.

3. Preheat the oven to 450 degrees F. Grease a shallow roasting pan.

4. In a large skillet, heat the remaining oil on medium heat. Add onion and remaining garlic and sauté for about 2-3 minutes.

5. Add kale and cook for about 8-10 minutes. Remove from heat and set aside to cool for at least 10 minutes. Stir in remaining ingredients.

6. Place the leg of lamb on a smooth surface, cut-side up. Place

the kale mixture in the center, leaving a 1-inch border from both sides.

7. Roll the short side to seal the stuffing. With a kitchen string, tightly tie the roll at many places. Arrange the roll into the prepared roasting pan, seam-side down. Roast for about 15 minutes.

8. Reduce the temperature of the oven to 350 degrees F. Roast for about 1-1¼ hours. Remove the lamb from the oven and set aside for about 10-20 minutes before slicing.

9. With a sharp knife, cut the roll into desired-sized slices and serve.

Nutritional Information Per Serving:

Calories: 350
Fat: 16.5g
Sat. Fat: 5.5g
Sodium: 245mg
Carbohydrates: 4g
Fiber: 0.7g
Sugar: 0.4g
Protein: 44.3g

Cheesy Tilapia

Yield: Makes 8 portions
Cooking Time: 5 minutes

Ingredients

½ cup Parmesan cheese, grated
3 tablespoons mayonnaise
¼ cup butter, softened
2 tablespoons fresh lemon juice
2 pounds tilapia fillets
¼ teaspoon dried thyme, crushed
Salt and freshly ground black pepper, to taste

Directions:

1. Preheat the broiler. Grease the broiler pan.

2. In a large bowl, mix all ingredients except the tilapia fillets. Set aside.

3. Place the fillets on the prepared broiler pan in a single layer. Broil the fillets for about 2-3 minutes. Remove from the oven and top the fillets evenly with cheese mixture.

4. Broil for about an additional 2 minutes.

Nutritional Information Per Serving:

Calories: 187
Fat: 10g
Sat. Fat: 5.3g
Sodium: 225mg
Carbohydrates: 1.6g
Fiber: 0g
Sugar: 0.4g
Protein: 23.1g

Cheesy Tilapia II

Yield: Makes 8 portions
Cooking Time: 23 minutes

Ingredients

1/3 cup mayonnaise
2 garlic cloves, minced
2 tablespoons fresh lemon juice
1 tablespoon Dijon mustard
2 pounds salmon fillet
1 large onion, sliced thinly
Salt and freshly ground black pepper, to taste
¼ cup Parmesan cheese, shredded finely
½ cup Mozzarella cheese, shredded finely

Directions:

1. Preheat the oven to 400 degrees F. Line a rimmed baking sheet with a piece of foil.

2. In a small bowl, combine the mayonnaise, lemon juice, mustard and garlic.

3. Arrange the salmon fillet onto the prepared baking sheet and sprinkle with salt and pepper. Place the onion slices evenly over the salmon fillets. Spread the mayonnaise mixture evenly over the onions. Top with the cheeses.

4. Bake for about 15-18 minutes. Set the oven to broiler. Broil the salmon fillets for about 2-5 minutes.

Nutritional Information Per Serving:

Calories: 327
Fat: 17.9g

Sat. Fat: 4.6g
Sodium: 459mg
Carbohydrates: 9.6g
Fiber: 0.7g
Sugar: 2g
Protein: 35.7g

Spinach Pie

Yield: Makes 5 portions
Cooking Time: 40 minutes

Ingredients

2 tablespoons butter, divided
2 tablespoons onion, chopped
1 (16-ounce) bag frozen chopped spinach, thawed and squeezed
1½ cups heavy cream
3 organic eggs
½ teaspoon ground nutmeg
Salt and freshly ground black pepper, to taste
½ cup swiss cheese, shredded

Directions:

1. Preheat the oven to 375 degrees F. Grease a 9-inch pie dish.

2. In a large skillet, melt 1 tablespoon of butter on medium-high heat.

3. Add onion and sauté for about 4-5 minutes. Add spinach and cook for about 2-3 minutes or until all the liquid is absorbed.

4. In a bowl, add cream, eggs, nutmeg, salt and black pepper and beat until well combined.

5. Transfer the spinach mixture evenly to the bottom of the prepared pie dish.

6. Place the egg mixture evenly over the spinach mixture. Sprinkle evenly with Swiss cheese.

7. Top with the remaining butter in the shape of dots at many places.

8. Bake for about 25-30 minutes or until the top becomes golden brown.

Nutritional Information Per Serving:

Calories: 599
Fat: 59.5g
Sat. Fat: 36.2g
Sodium: 243mg
Carbohydrates: 8.2g
Fiber: 2.2g
Sugar: 1.1g
Protein: 11.6g

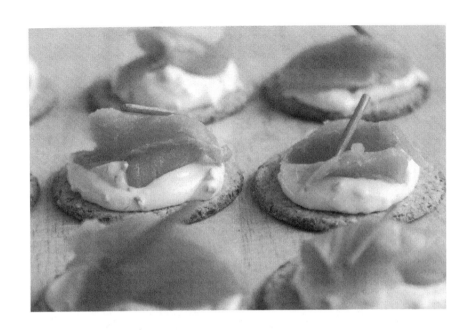

KETO SNACKS

Cinnamon Cookies

Yield: Makes 15 cookies (1 cookie per serving)
Cooking Time: 25 minutes

Ingredients

2 cups almond meal
1 teaspoon ground cinnamon
1 organic egg
½ cup salted butter, softened
1 teaspoon liquid stevia
1 teaspoon vanilla extract

Directions:

1. Preheat the oven to 300 degrees F. Grease a large cookie sheet.

2. In a large bowl, add all ingredients and mix until well combined. Make 15 equal-sized balls.

3. Arrange the balls onto the prepared baking sheet about 2 inches apart. Bake for about 5 minutes.

4. Remove the cookie sheet from the oven and, with a fork, press down on each ball. Bake for about 18-20 minutes.

5. Remove from the oven and set onto the wire rack to cool in the pan for about 5 minutes.

6. Carefully invert the cookies onto the wire rack to cool completely before serving.

Nutritional Information Per Serving:

Calories: 133
Fat: 12.8g
Sat. Fat: 4.5g
Sodium: 48mg

Carbohydrates: 2.9g
Fiber: 1.7g
Sugar: 0.6g
Protein: 3.1g

Cheese Biscuits

Yield: Makes 8 biscuits (1 biscuit per serving)
Cooking Time: 15 minutes

Ingredients

1/3 cup coconut flour, sifted
¼ teaspoon baking powder
Salt, to taste
4 organic eggs
¼ cup butter, melted and cooled
1 cup cheddar cheese, shredded

Directions:

1. Preheat the oven to 400 degrees F. Line a large cookie sheet with a greased piece of foil.

2. In a large bowl, mix flour, baking powder, garlic powder and salt.

3. In another bowl, add eggs and butter and beat well. Add egg mixture to flour mixture and beat until well combined. Fold in cheese.

4. With a tablespoon, place the mixture onto prepared cookie sheets in a single layer.

5. Bake for about 15 minutes or until the top becomes golden brown.

Nutritional Information Per Serving:

Calories:142
Fat: 12.7g
Sat. Fat: 7.4g
Sodium: 180mg

Carbohydrates: 0.8g
Fiber: 0.2g
Sugar: 0.3g
Protein:

Celery Crackers

Yield: Makes 15 portions
Cooking Time: 2 hours

Ingredients

10 celery stalks
1 teaspoon fresh rosemary leaves
1 teaspoon fresh thyme leaves
2 tablespoons raw apple cider vinegar
¼ cup avocado oil
Salt, to taste
3 cups flax seeds, ground roughly

Directions:

1. Preheat the oven to 225 degrees F. Line 2 large baking sheets with parchment paper.

2. In a food processor, add all ingredients except flax seeds and pulse until a puree forms.

3. Add flax seeds and pulse until well combined. Transfer the dough into a bowl and set aside for about 2-3 minutes. Divide the dough into 2 portions.

4. Place 1 portion evenly in each prepared baking sheets.

5. With the back of a spatula, smooth and press the dough to ¼-inch thickness.

6. With a knife, score squares in the dough. Bake for about 1 hour. Flip and bake for 1 hour more.

7. Remove from the oven and set aside to cool on the baking sheet for about 15 minutes.

Nutritional Information Per Serving:

Calories: 126
Fat: 7.6g
Sat. Fat: 1.1g
Sodium: 27mg
Carbohydrates: 7.1g
Fiber: 6.5g
Sugar: 0.5g
Protein: 4.3g

Zucchini Sticks

Yield: Makes 8 portions
Cooking Time: 25 minutes

Ingredients

2 zucchinis, cut lengthwise into 3-inch sticks
Salt, to taste
2 organic eggs
½ cup Parmesan cheese, grated
½ cup almonds, grounded
½ teaspoon Italian herb seasoning

Directions:

1. Place the zucchini sticks in a large colander and sprinkle with salt. Set aside for about 1 hour to drain.

2. Preheat the oven to 425 degrees F. Line a large baking sheet with parchment paper.

3. Squeeze the zucchini sticks to remove excess liquid. With a paper towel, pat dry the zucchini sticks.

4. In a shallow dish, crack the eggs and beat. In another shallow dish, mix the remaining ingredients.

5. Dip the zucchini sticks in egg and then coat evenly with the cheese mixture.

6. Arrange the zucchini sticks in the prepared baking sheet in a single layer. Bake for about 25 minutes, turning once halfway through.

Nutritional Information Per Serving:

Calories: 133
Fat: 9.2g

Sat. Fat: 3.1g
Sodium: 281mg
Carbohydrates: 4.5g
Fiber: 1.7g
Sugar: 1.6g
Protein: 9.4g

Devilled Eggs

Yield: Makes 6 portions
Cooking Time: 5 minutes

Ingredients

6 organic eggs
¼ cup mayonnaise
¼ onion, chopped finely
½ celery stalk, chopped finely
Drop of hot sauce
Pinch of salt
Pinch of paprika

Directions:

1. In a large pan of water, add eggs and bring to a boil on high heat.

2. Cover the pan and immediately remove from heat. Set aside, covered, for at least 10-12 minutes.

3. Drain the water and set aside to cool completely. Peel the eggs, then cut in half lengthwise.

4. Remove the egg yolks and place in a bowl. Add the remaining ingredients except the paprika and stir to combine.

5. Place the celery mixture evenly in the egg white halves. Sprinkle with paprika.

6. Arrange the eggs on a plate. Cover and chill before serving.

Nutritional Information Per Serving:

Calories: 107
Fat: 7.7g

Sat. Fat: 1.8g
Sodium: 168mg
Carbohydrates: 3.5g
Fiber: 0.1g
Sugar: 1.5g
Protein: 5.7g

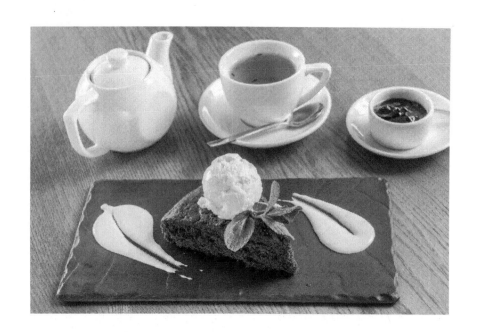

KETOGENIC DESSERTS

Pumpkin Custard

Yield: Makes 6 portions
Cooking Time: 50 minutes

Ingredients

1 (15-ounce) can pumpkin puree
4 organic eggs, beaten
½ cup heavy cream
2 teaspoons vanilla extract
1 teaspoon cinnamon liquid stevia
2 teaspoons pumpkin pie spice
¼ teaspoon salt

Directions:

1. Preheat the oven to 350 degrees F. Grease 6 ramekins.

2. In a large bowl, add all ingredients and beat until smooth.

3. Transfer the mixture evenly into the prepared ramekins. Bake for about 45-50 minutes or until a knife inserted in the center comes out clean.

4. Serve warm.

Nutritional Information Per Serving:

Calories: 107
Fat: 6.9g
Sat. Fat: 3.4g
Sodium: 146mg
Carbohydrates: 6.8g
Fiber: 2.1g
Sugar: 2.8g
Protein: 4.7g

Blueberry Cobbler

Yield: Makes 10 portions
Cooking Time: 22 minutes

Ingredients

For Filling

3 cups fresh blueberries
2 tablespoons Swerve
¼ teaspoon xanthan gum
1 teaspoon fresh lemon juice

For Topping:

2/3 cup almond flour
2 tablespoons Swerve
2 tablespoons butter, melted
½ teaspoon fresh lemon zest, grated finely

Directions:

1. Preheat the oven to 375 degrees F.

2. For filling in a bowl, mix all ingredients. Transfer the mixture into a 9x9-inch pie dish.

3. In another bowl, add all topping ingredients and mix until a crumbly mixture forms.

4. Place the topping mixture evenly over the blueberry mixture.

5. Bake for about 22 minutes or until the top becomes golden brown.

6. Serve

Nutritional Information Per Serving:

Calories: 57
Fat: 3.4g
Sat. Fat: 1.5g
Sodium: 146mg
Carbohydrates: 13.1g
Fiber: 1.6g
Sugar: 10.4g
Protein: 0.8g

Lemon Mousse

Yield: Makes 5 portions

Ingredients

¼ cup fresh lemon juice
8 ounces cream cheese, softened
1 cup heavy cream
1/8 teaspoon salt
½-1 teaspoon lemon liquid stevia

Directions:

1. In a blender, add lemon juice and cream cheese and pulse until smooth.

2. Add remaining ingredients and pulse until well combined and fluffy.

3. Transfer the mixture into serving glasses. Refrigerate to chill before serving.

Nutritional Information Per Serving:

Calories: 244
Fat: 24.8g
Sat. Fat: 15.6g
Sodium: 204mg
Carbohydrates: 2.1g
Fiber: 0.1g
Sugar: 0.4g
Protein: 4g

Frozen Yogurt

Yield: Makes 6 portions

Ingredients

3 cups plain Greek yogurt
3-4 drops liquid stevia
1 teaspoon vanilla extract

Directions:

1. In a bowl, add all ingredients and mix until well combined.

2. Transfer the mixture into an ice cream maker and process according to the manufacturer's directions.

3. Transfer the mixture into a bowl. Cover and freeze for about 30-40 minutes or until the desired consistency is reached.

Nutritional Information Per Serving:

Calories: 89
Fat: 1.5g
Sat. Fat: 1.2g
Sodium: 86mg
Carbohydrates: 8.7g
Fiber: 0g
Sugar: 8.7g
Protein: 7g

Zucchini Brownies

Yield: Makes 20 portions
Cooking Time: 45 minutes

Ingredients

1½ cups zucchini, shredded
1 cup dark chocolate chips
1 organic egg
1 cup butter
1/3 cup unsweetened applesauce
1 teaspoon vanilla extract
1 teaspoon baking soda
1 teaspoon ground cinnamon
½ teaspoon ground nutmeg

Directions:

1. Preheat the oven to 350 degrees F. Grease a 9x9-inch baking dish.

2. In a large bowl, add all ingredients and mix until well combined.

3. Transfer the mixture evenly into the prepared baking dish. With the back of a spatula, smooth the top surface.

4. Bake for about 35-45 minutes or until a toothpick inserted in the center comes out clean.

5. Remove from the oven and set aside to cool completely. After cooling, cut into desired-sized squares and serve.

Nutritional Information Per Serving:

Calories: 117
Fat: 11.1g

Sat. Fat: 6.9g
Sodium: 132mg
Carbohydrates: 4.9g
Fiber: 0.2g
Sugar: 3.8g
Protein: 0.9g

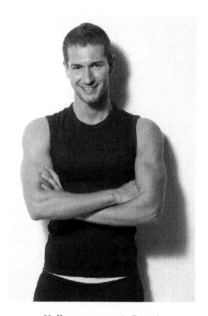

Hello, my name is Dave!

I hope you like my books. Let me tell you a little about myself.

For 7 years now I have been working as a personal fitness trainer. During this time, I realized that it is not enough just to make an effective training plan. Training in the hall is only a small part of the work on the way to a healthy, strong and beautiful body. In my opinion, the formula looks like this: 30% training, 30% an active way of life and positive thinking, and 40% healthy eating. I like to cook, I love to write, and I like to invent recipes. All my knowledge and passion were embodied in my books. There is a huge variety of diets that allow you to quickly lose weight. I'm not sure they are all useful. In my books, I write about diets that not only lead to weight loss, but also give health and vivacity. I hope they will benefit you, too!

Be sure to subscribe to the newsletter to receive news of new books and bonuses from me.

With love,

Dave

Find my books on Amazon!

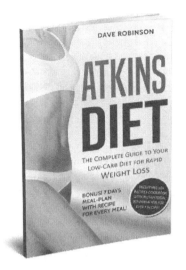 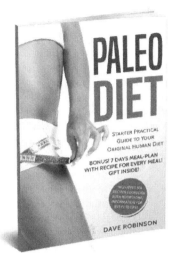

amazon.com/author/dave.robinson

Please leave feedback if you love them!

It is very important for me

Made in the USA
San Bernardino, CA
10 March 2018